Cooking With Veggie Vero

A children's recipe book of simple plant-based snacks

Veronica Green

Cooking With Veggie Vero
ISBN 978-1-7354121-3-9

Veronica Green Publications

Author's Note

As a writer and activist, my mission is to empower children with the skills to live consciously and compassionately. I believe that a kind and sustainable future begins with a generation of young environmentalists who understand the ripple effects of their daily choices. Cooking with organic, plant-based foods helps to nurture a deep appreciation for the Earth's abundance.
This opens the door for family discussions about how we can protect our planet.

My heart is filled with gratitude for having been given the opportunity to educate children and families about plant based foods. Leading the cooking segment of the Nature Education Cooperative at the Delray Beach Children's Garden has been such a rewarding experience. The children with their inquisitive minds, boundless creativity and instinctive connection to nature, have taught me so very much. I've come to understand that the more I teach, the more I learn. What a beautiful cycle!

This book is a collection of recipes that have been most popular with my students. The more involved children are in the cooking process, the more open they become to trying new things.

I encourage you to release the notion that food (and art) needs to look a certain way. Allow your child to experiment with the various shapes and textures of new foods. The end result is not nearly as important as the process!

I hope this book will inspire many creative cooking sessions in your home. The recipes are all plant-based and can be easily modified for gluten-free and nut-free preferences. Happy cooking!

- Veronica Green

Tips For Preparation

* Use organic ingredients whenever possible! Have discussions about the benefits of organic and locally grown produce.

* Throughout this book, my portion sizes will be for one child. Modify quantities to meet your needs!

* I love using 6-count cupcake tins as a serving platter for ingredients. The separated cups are the perfect size for holding small portions of raw ingredients.

* Be sure to provide young chefs with all the materials needed for their cooking session. This will often include a cutting board, a mixing bowl, a serving plate for the finished product, and utensils.

* Some recipes will call for pre-cooked ingredients (rice or quinoa, for example). If you want to involve your young chef in the slower cooking process, that's wonderful! For eager young chefs (often 5 years or younger), you may decide to have those items cooked in advance, so they can dive right in to the fun part!

Lettuce Begin!

Loaded Avocado Toast

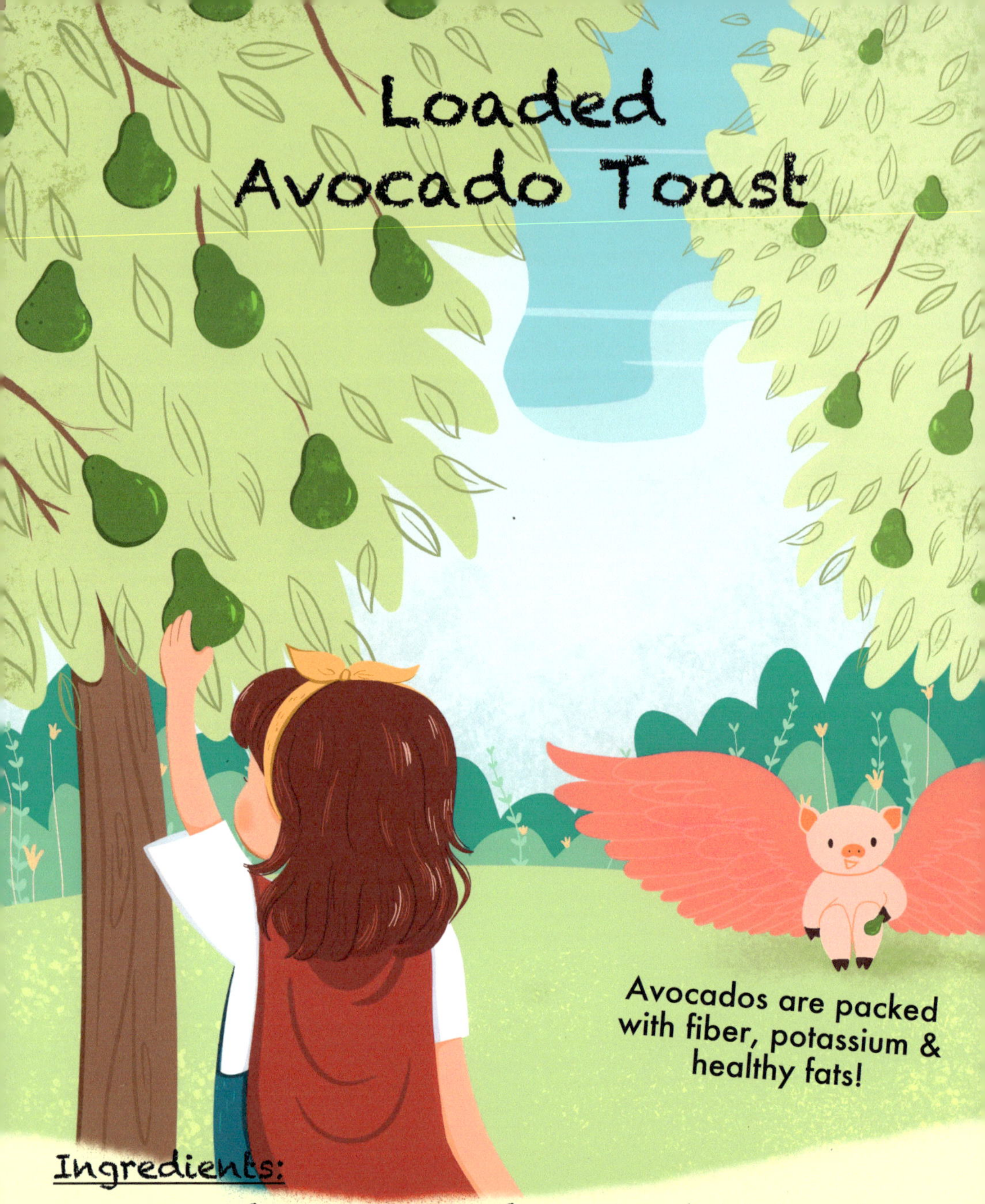

Avocados are packed with fiber, potassium & healthy fats!

Ingredients:

- 2 slices of your choice of Bread (Substitute with crackers, pita or flatbread, if desired!)
- 1/2 a ripe Avocado
- 1 wedge of Lime
- 1/2 cup of Garbanzo Beans
- 3 to 6 Cherry Tomatoes
- "Everything" seasoning to taste (or salt & pepper)
- Fresh Dill (or Cilantro)

Steps:

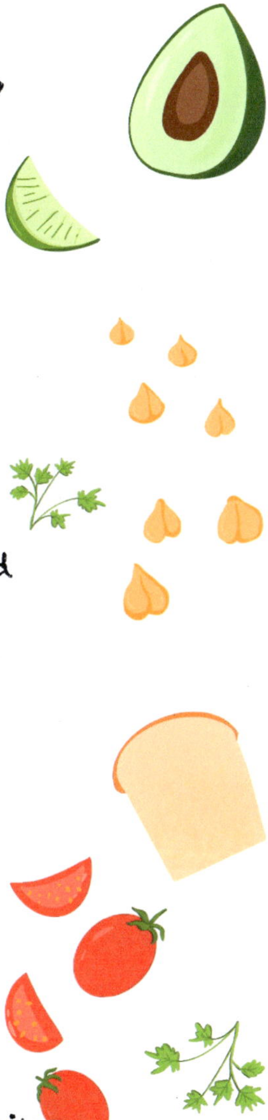

1. Using a fork, mash your avocado into a mixing bowl.
2. Add lime juice and garbanzo beans into your bowl. Mix it up!
3. Chop your tomatoes. You can either add them to your mixture now, or save them for later to create funny shapes on your toast :)
4. Sprinkle some "Everything" seasoning into your mixture. You can substitute with salt & pepper if needed!
5. Toast your bread. (Alternatives to bread can be crackers, pita or flatbread!)
6. Spread a thick layer of your avocado mixture onto the toast. Add tomatoes on top, if you didn't already.
7. Chop up your dill or cilantro. It's ok to break it apart with your hands! Sprinkle it onto your toast.
8. If desired, top it off with a little more 'Everything' seasoning. Enjoy!

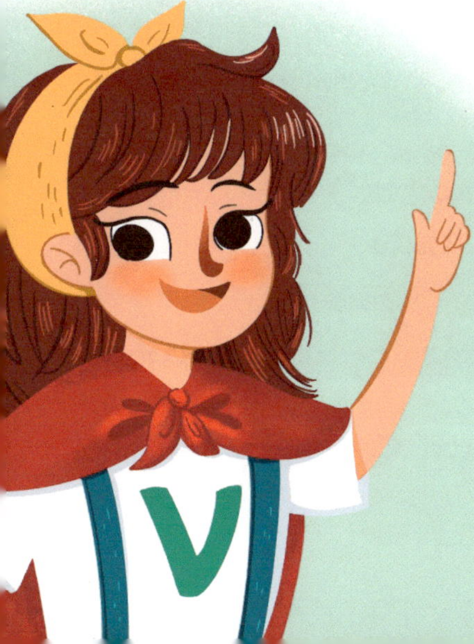

Note:
'Everything' seasoning is made of salt, dried garlic & onion powder, poppy seeds and sesame seeds. You can make it, or buy it pre-made in most markets near the seasonings!

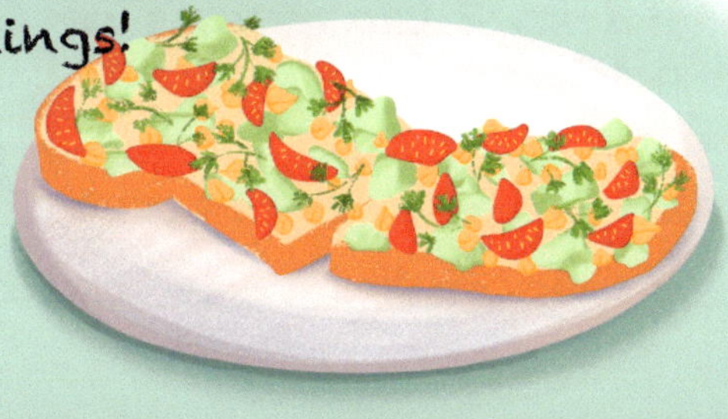

No-Bake Energy Bites

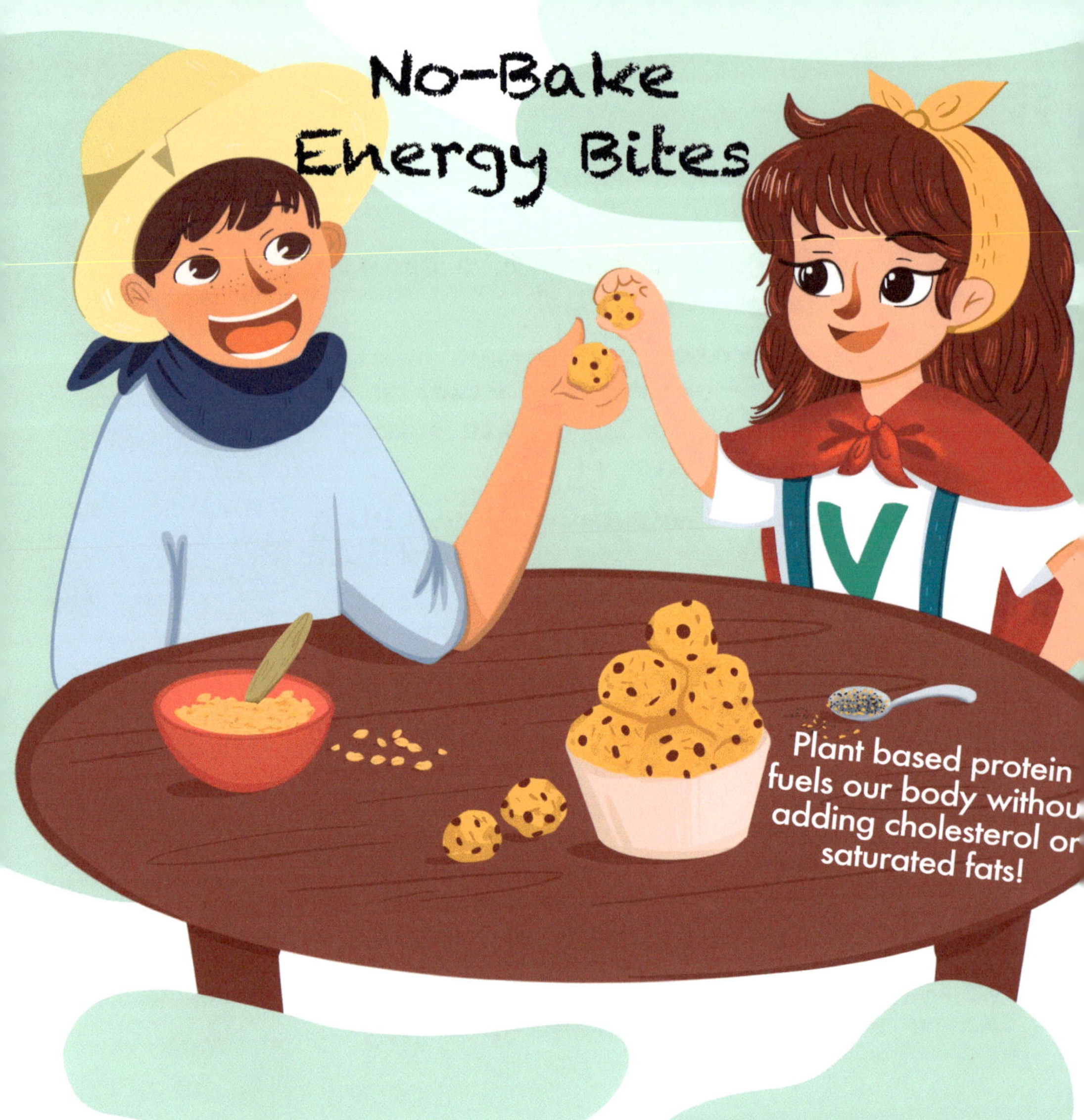

Ingredients: *makes about 4 energy bites

- 1 heaping tablespoon of any Nut or Seed Butter (I recommend Sunflower Seed Butter!)
- 3 tablespoons of dry Rolled Oats
- 2 teaspoons of organic Maple Syrup
- 1 to 2 teaspoons of Chia seeds (optional, but adds great nutritional value!)
- 2 teaspoons of Dark Chocolate Chips, Cacao Nibs or Raisins (optional)
- Coconut shreds (optional)

Steps:

1. Add your nut or seed butter along with the dry rolled oats and maple syrup into a mixing bowl.
2. Use a spoon to mix it up until you have a nice thick mixture. This is your base! If you find it is too dry, add a little bit more maple. If it seems too slimy, add more oats to absorb the moisture.
3. Add your optional extras into the mixture. (chia seeds/chocolate chips/raisins/coconut shreds) Mix it up!
4. Once your mixture is just right, use your clean hands to roll out bite-sized energy balls.
5. If using coconut, you may want to roll your energy balls onto a plate of coconut shreds and shake off any loose shreds.
6. Enjoy at room temperature, or refrigerate for 30 to 40 minutes. Refrigerating helps to bind the mixture and makes for a cleaner bite. Yummy!

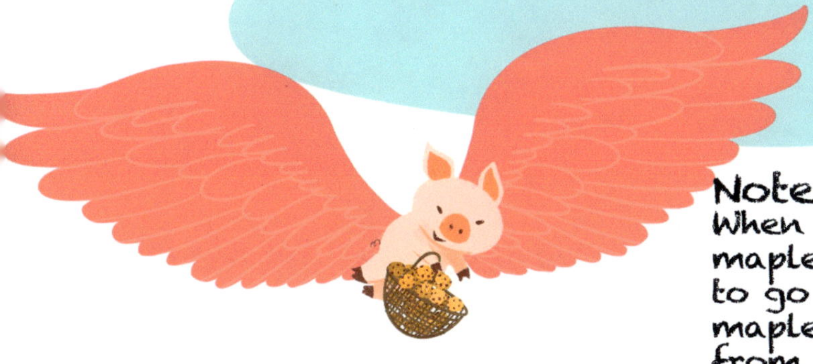

Note:
When selecting a maple syrup, be sure to go for pure 100% maple. It comes from a maple tree. There should be no other ingredients!

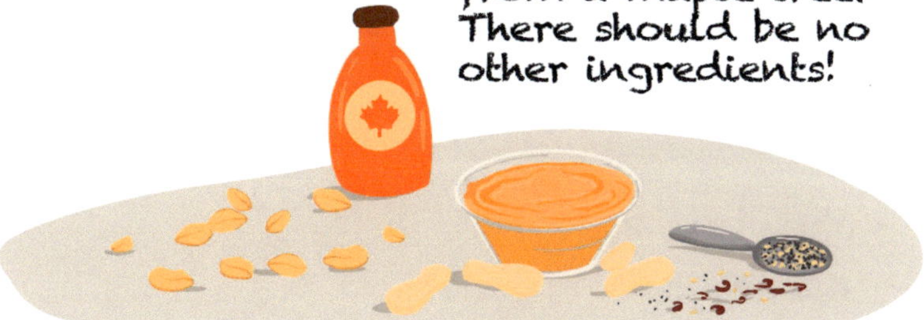

Rainbow Lettuce Wraps

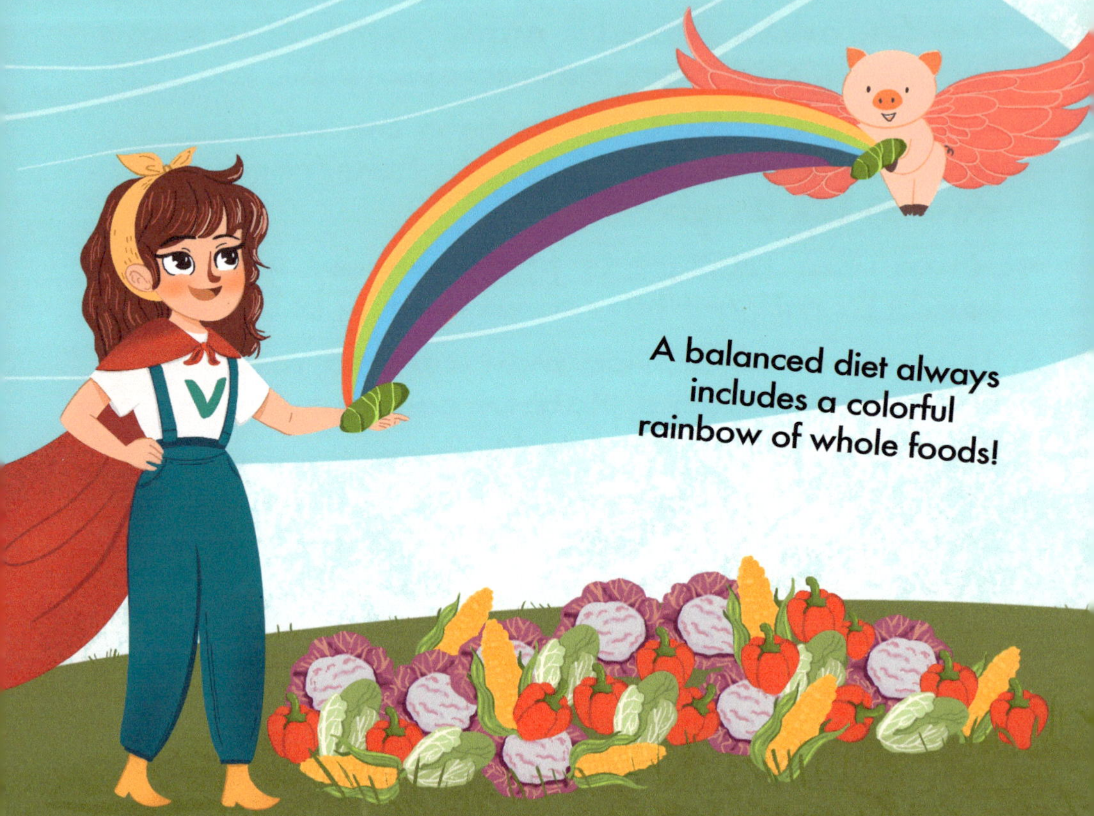

Ingredients:

- large leafy Greens
(I recommend collard greens! Other options are romaine, bib, or butter head lettuce.)
- Red Bell Pepper
- Orange Carrots (preferably shredded)
- Sweet Corn (canned or cob. May substitute with any other yellow produce such as pineapple or bell pepper)
- Purple Cabbage
- Hummus

Steps:

1. Cut the stem off your leafy green so it lays flat. Some lettuce won't lay flat (like Romaine), so it will be more of a lettuce taco, but that's okay! If using a collard green, you may choose to blanch it in hot water for a few seconds to soften it. That's optional, raw is fine!
2. Use a spoon to spread a layer of hummus all over one side of your leafy green.
3. Chop up your ingredients. There's no wrong way! Long strips or little chunks... it will still be tasty!
4. Arrange your chopped veggies onto the wrap in rows of color. Is it looking like a rainbow?
5. Roll it up, using the hummus as a paste to seal it closed. You can also use a toothpick to secure it!
6. If your finished wrap has floppy ends, you might want to use a knife or kitchen scissor to cut about an inch off from each end. This ensures the first bite will be full of rainbow goodness. Enjoy!

Note:
You can easily make your own hummus by blending chickpeas, tahini, garlic, lemon, cumin and salt. Blend until creamy.

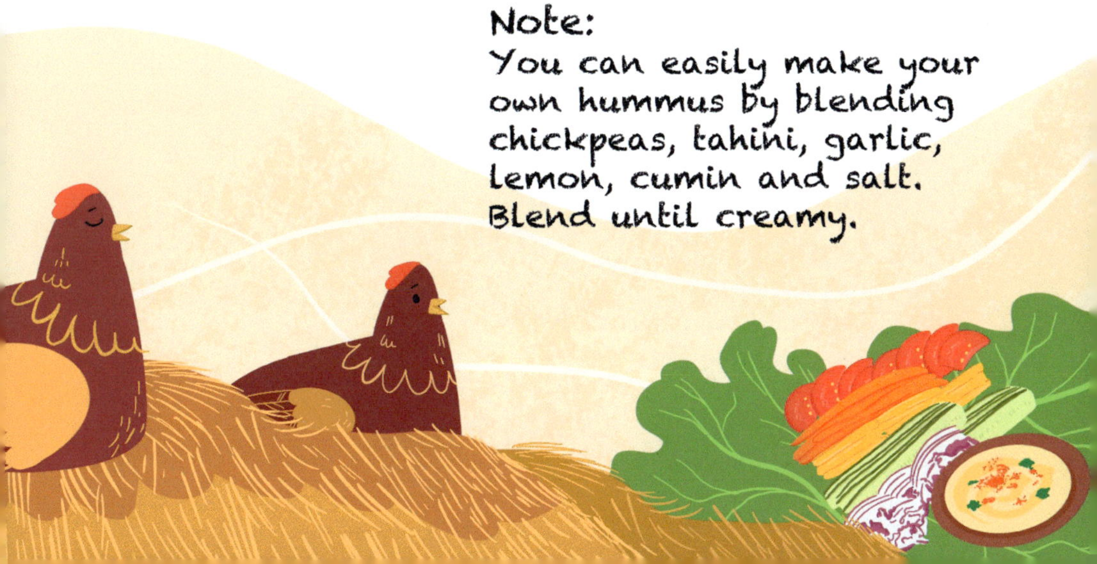

Teriyaki Veggie Skewers

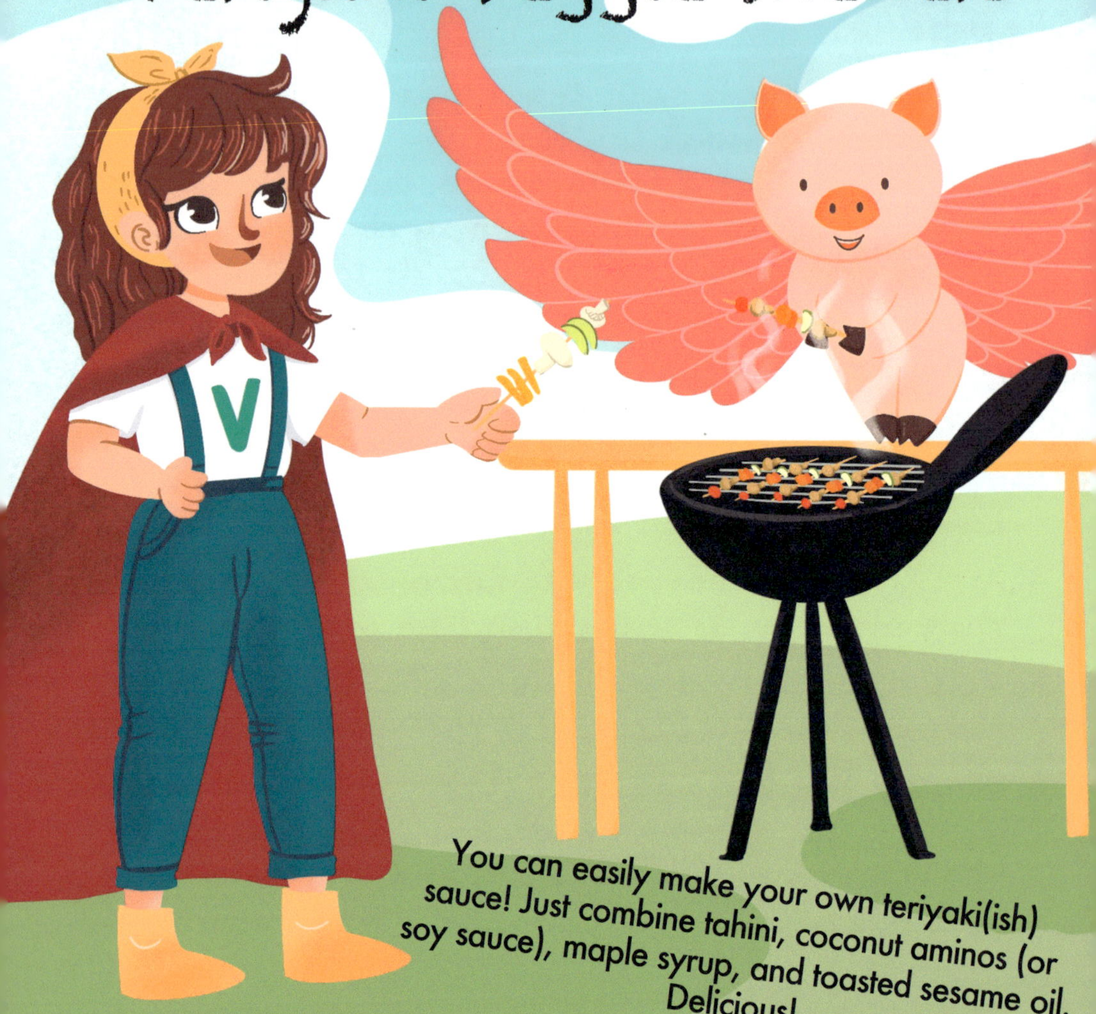

You can easily make your own teriyaki(ish) sauce! Just combine tahini, coconut aminos (or soy sauce), maple syrup, and toasted sesame oil. Delicious!

Ingredients:

- Teriyaki Sauce
- Cherry Tomatoes
- Pineapple
- Mushrooms
- Firm Tofu
- Green Bell Pepper (and/or Zucchini)

*This recipe requires some heat. If using a stove top, I recommend a wide, square-shaped pan and short skewer sticks. This allows the skewer to lay flat while cooking.

Steps:

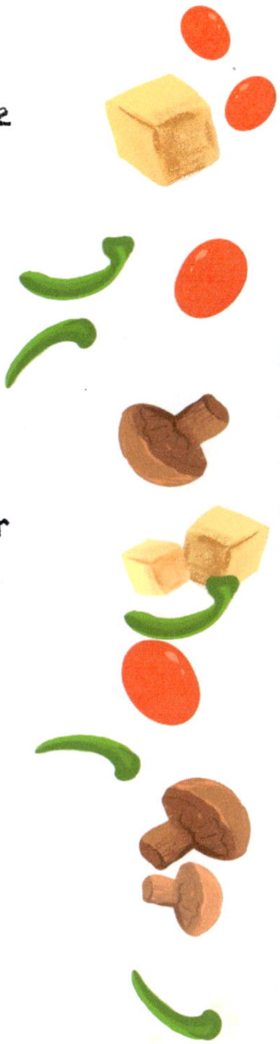

1. Chop your ingredients into chunks that are large enough to be pierced without falling apart. Cherry tomatoes can be left whole.
2. Begin piercing your ingredients onto the skewer. Have fun with the variety of patterns you can make!
3. Turn your grill or stove top on to a Low heat.
4. With an adult present, carefully place your skewers into the heat and slather on some teriyaki sauce.
5. Tend to your skewers patiently, rotating them every minute or so until desired browning is reached. Enjoy!!

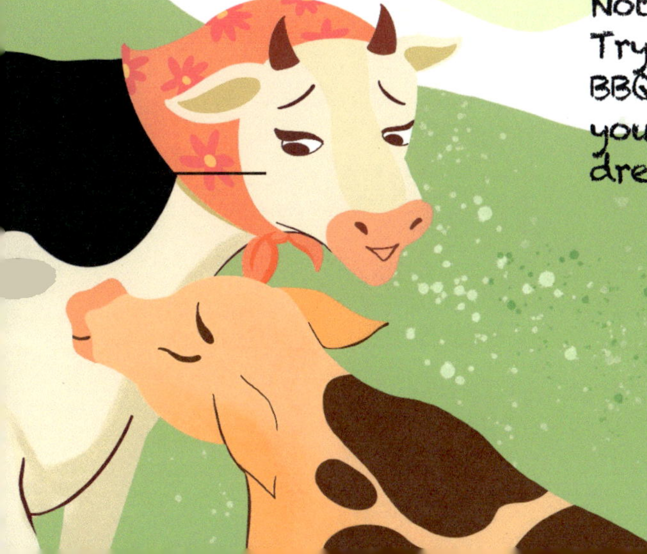

Note:

Not a fan of teriyaki? Try this recipe with BBQ sauce or even your favorite salad dressing!

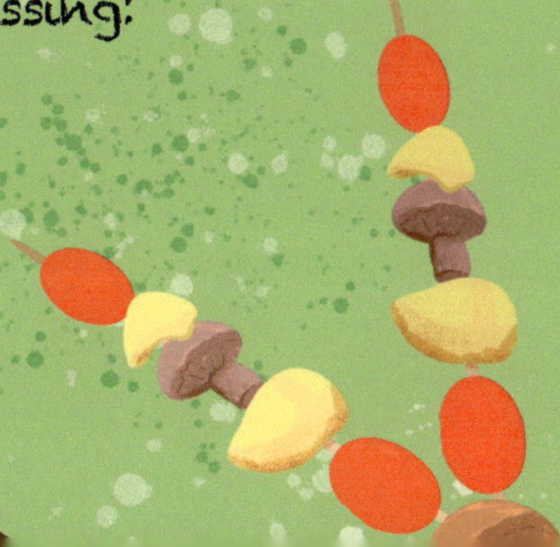

Zoodle Pesto

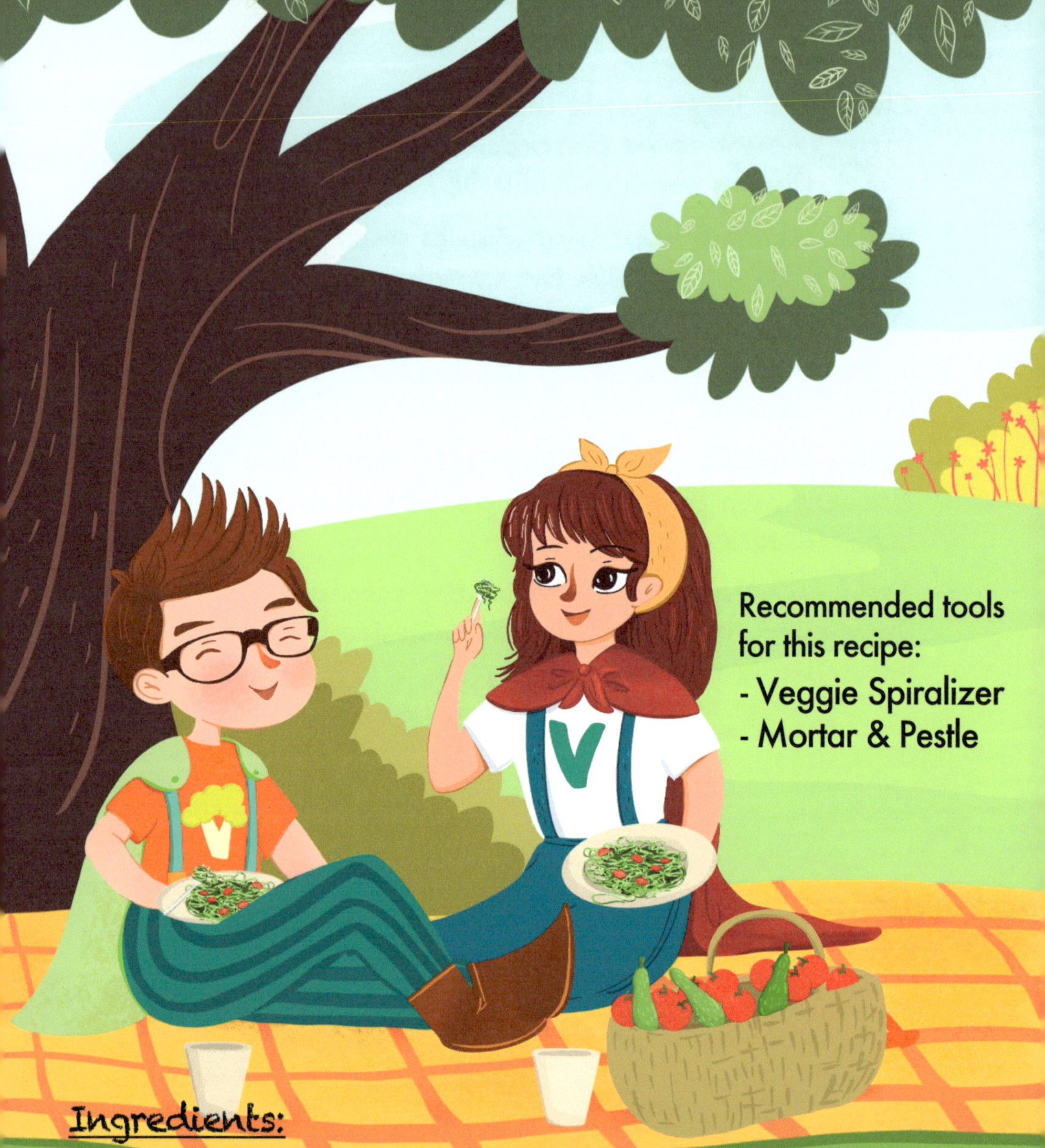

Recommended tools for this recipe:

- Veggie Spiralizer
- Mortar & Pestle

Ingredients:

- 1/2 a raw Zucchini
- 3 to 5 Cherry Tomatoes
- 2 cups fresh Basil (or 1 cup basil, 1 cup spinach)
- 3 tablespoons Olive Oil
- 1 tablespoon Lemon juice (add more if desired)
- 1 teaspoon Garlic Powder
- 1/4 teaspoon of Salt (add more if desired)
- 1 tablespoon of Pine Nuts (or sunflower seeds)
- 1/2 tablespoon Nutritional Yeast & Hemp Seeds (optional)

Steps:

1. Create your zucchini noodles using either a spiralizer (recommended), a mandolin or a potato peeler. Place your raw zoodles into a serving bowl!
2. Chop your tomatoes and add them to the serving bowl.
3. Time to make the pesto! (Without a blender) Place your bundle of fresh basil (and spinach, if you choose) onto the cutting board. Ball it up with your hands and use a knife to chop it well... Really well!
4. Place your chopped greens into a mortar bowl along with your oil, lemon, and seasonings.
5. Use the pestle to grind them well, releasing the basil's flavor.
6. Toss your pine nuts or sunflower seeds into the mortar and grind some more. This adds a yummy crunch! Now you have pesto! Does it smell delicious? Adjust seasonings, if needed.
7. Pour the pesto on top of the zucchini noodles and enjoy! Zoodle Pesto! (You can saute this in a pan, if desired. But raw is perfectly fine!)

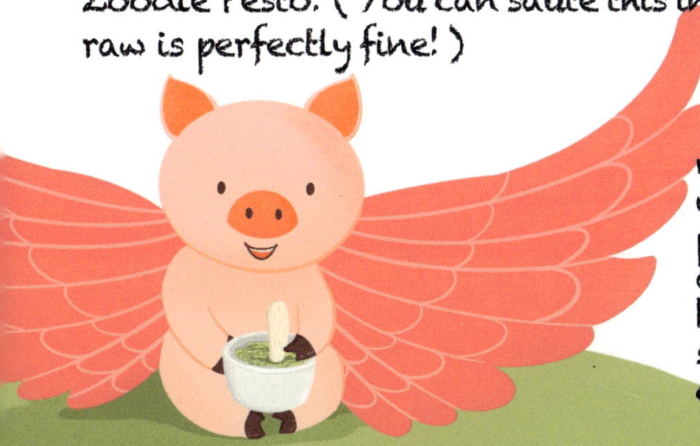

Note:

If you don't have a mortar & pestle, you can use a blender or food processor. However, the act of grinding food by hand is a fine-motor skill for kids & connects us to our meal!

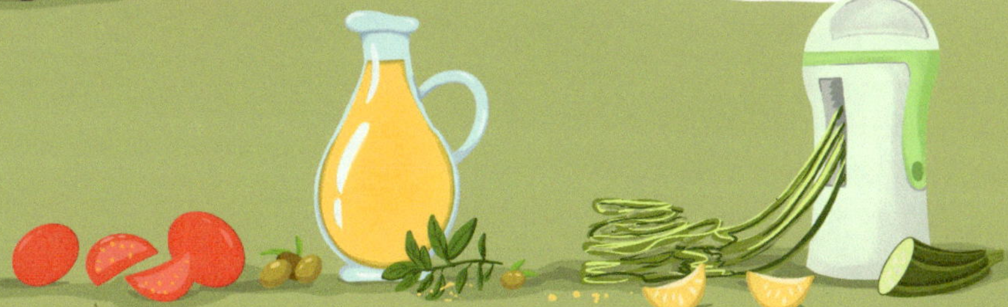

Mango Salsa

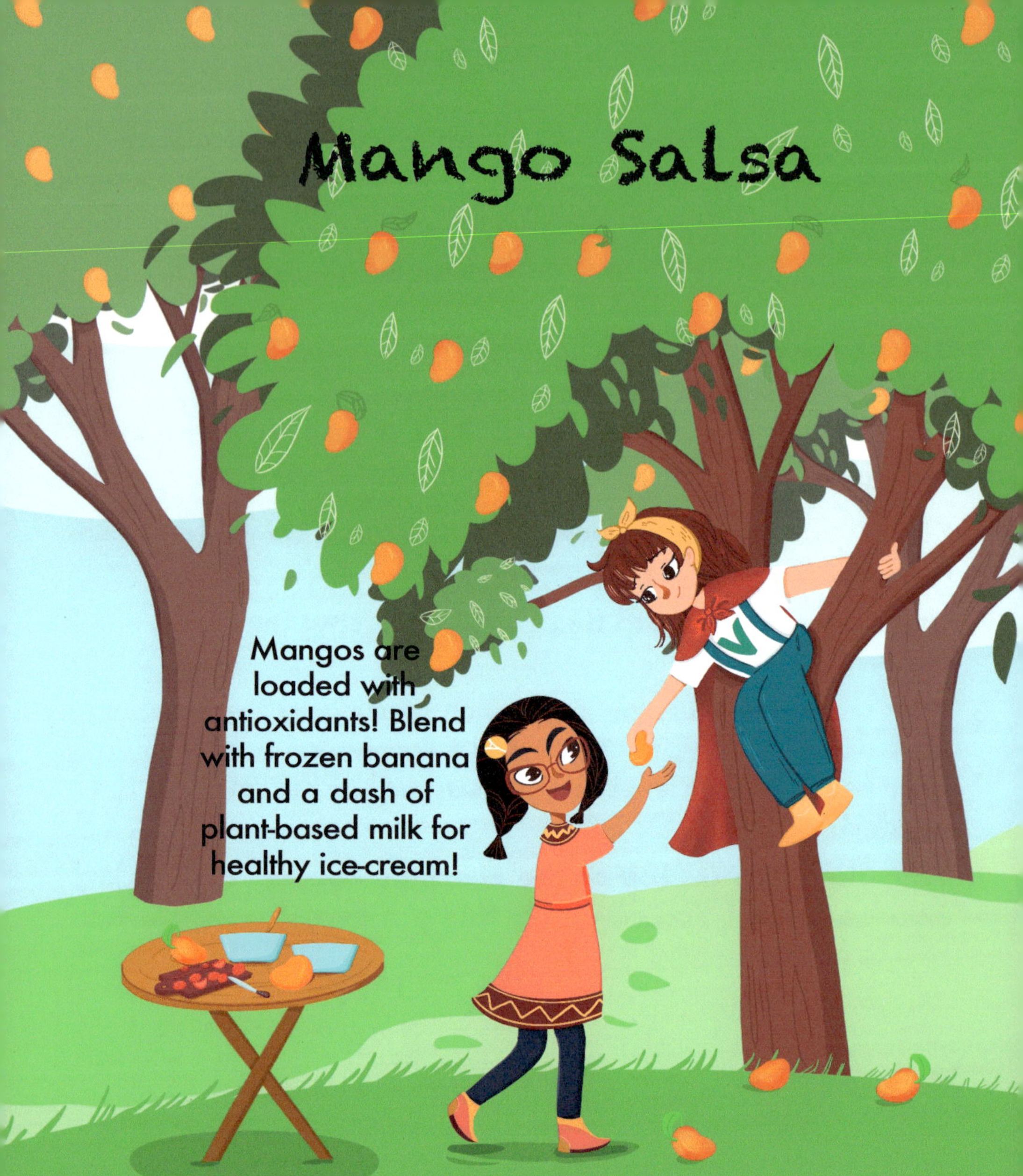

Mangos are loaded with antioxidants! Blend with frozen banana and a dash of plant-based milk for healthy ice-cream!

Ingredients:

- 1 Ripe Mango (Mango allergy? Use pineapple or even peaches instead!)
- 1/2 a Red Bell Pepper
- 1/2 a Plump Tomato (or 7 to 10 cherry tomatoes)
- 1/4 cup Fresh Cilantro Leaves
- Juice from 1/2 a Lime
- Pink Himalayan Salt to taste
- 1/4 cup Red Onion (you can substitute with green onions/scallions, which are easier on the eyes)

Steps:

1. Chop your mango and tomatoes into small bite-sized chunks on a cutting board. Add them to a mixing bowl. (be sure to scrape the juices into the bowl as well!)
2. Chop your bell pepper, onion, and cilantro next. Add it to the bowl! (Cilantro is often easier to break apart with your hands!)
3. Juice your lime right into the bowl, picking out any seeds that drop.
4. Add salt to taste.
5. Mix it all up and enjoy with your favorite chips!

Note:
To reduce tearing when cutting onions, chill onions for 30 minutes then cut off the top and peel outer layers, leaving the root end in tact. The root end contains the most sulphuric compounds!

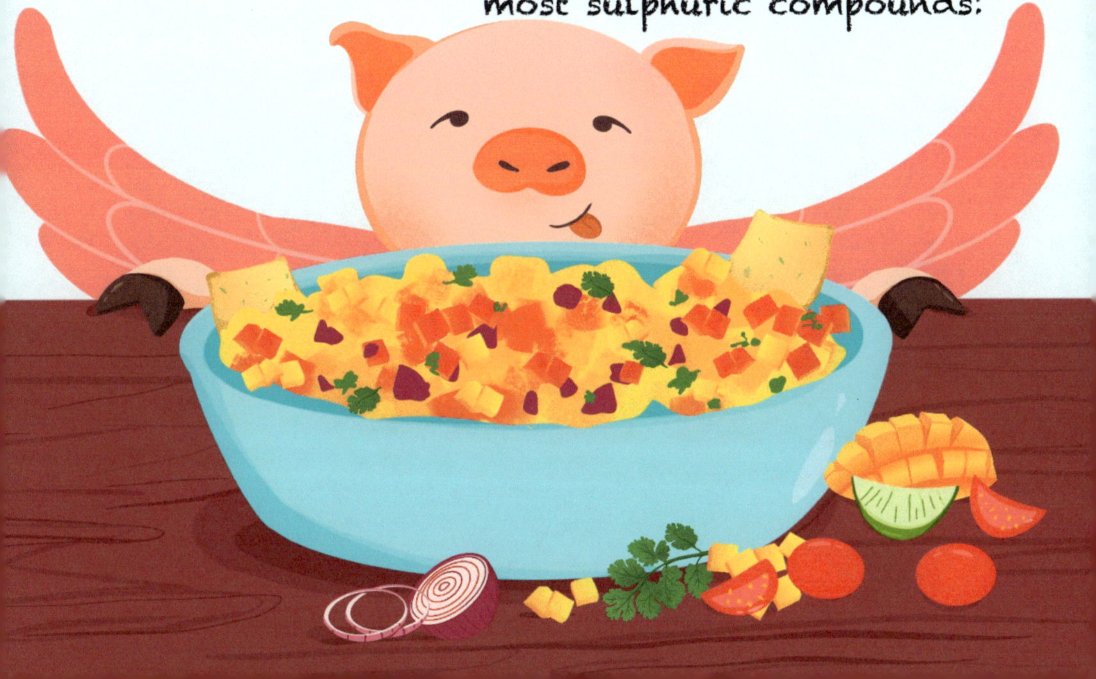

Cucumber Boats with Red Bean Pate

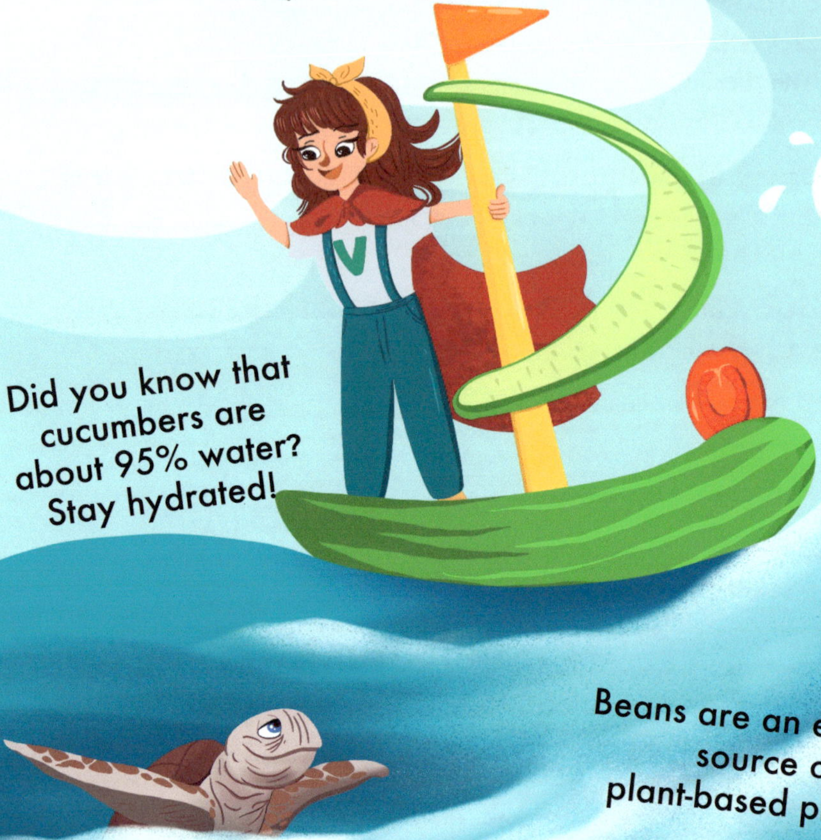

Ingredients:

- Cucumber
- 1/2 cup of Red Kidney Beans
- 2 Tablespoons of Tahini
- 1/4 Teaspoon of Salt
- 1/4 Teaspoon of Garlic Powder
- a pinch of Black Pepper (to taste)
- 1/2 Teaspoon of Maple Syrup
- a sprig of Fresh Cilantro (or parsley)

Steps:

1. Slice your cucumber into long strips. These will be your "boats." If desired, you can cut the cucumber in in half first, to create shorter boats. Don't slice them too thin, you'll need them to be sturdy!
2. Using a fork and a mixing bowl, mash your red beans, tahini and maple into a paste.
3. Add the salt, pepper and garlic powder. Mix it all up! Taste test it and adjust seasonings if needed.
4. Add the mixture onto your cucumber boats and top it off with fresh cilantro, if desired. Enjoy!

Note: Want to make a fun sail for your boat? Thinly slice half a cucumber (long ways) and bend it like the letter "C" Then stick a toothpick through it and add to your boat!

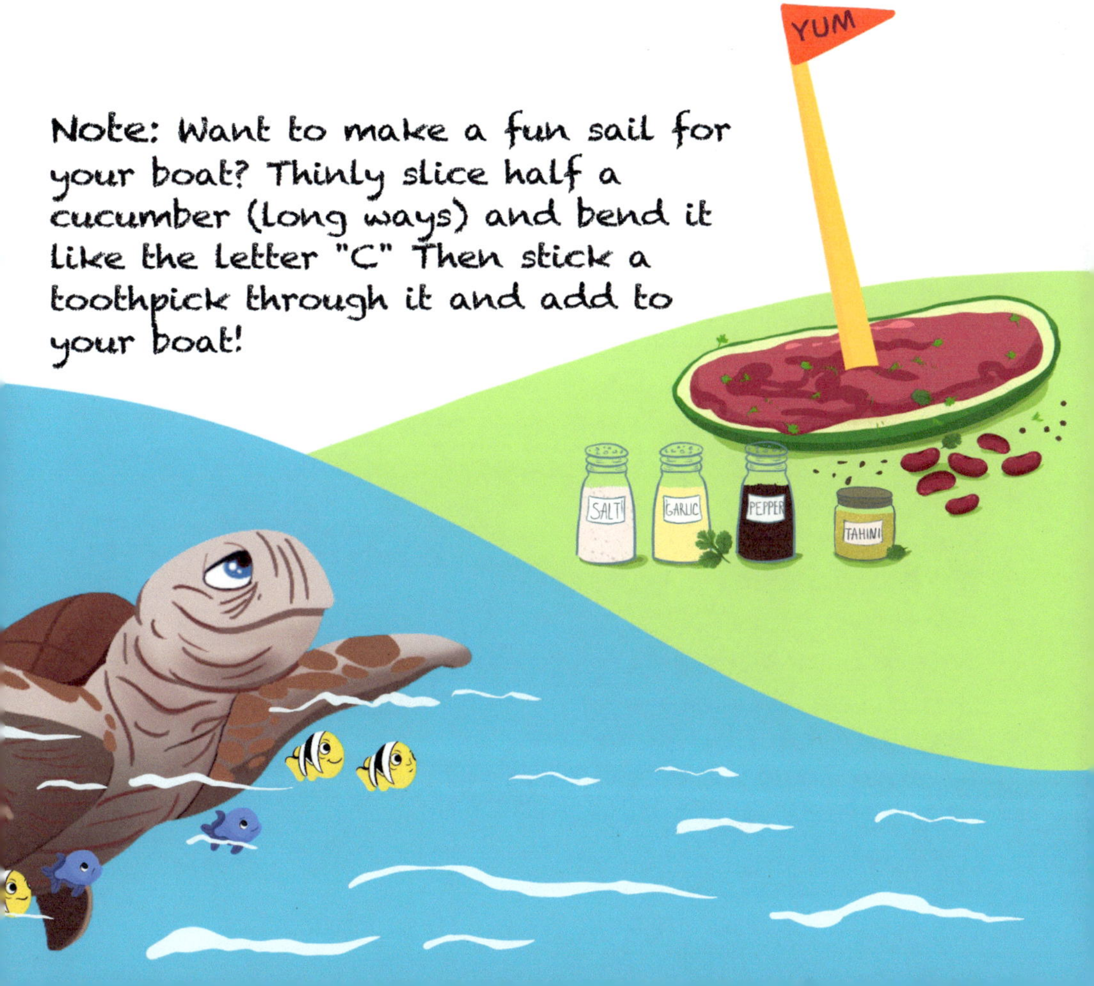

Raw Broccoli Salad in a Jar

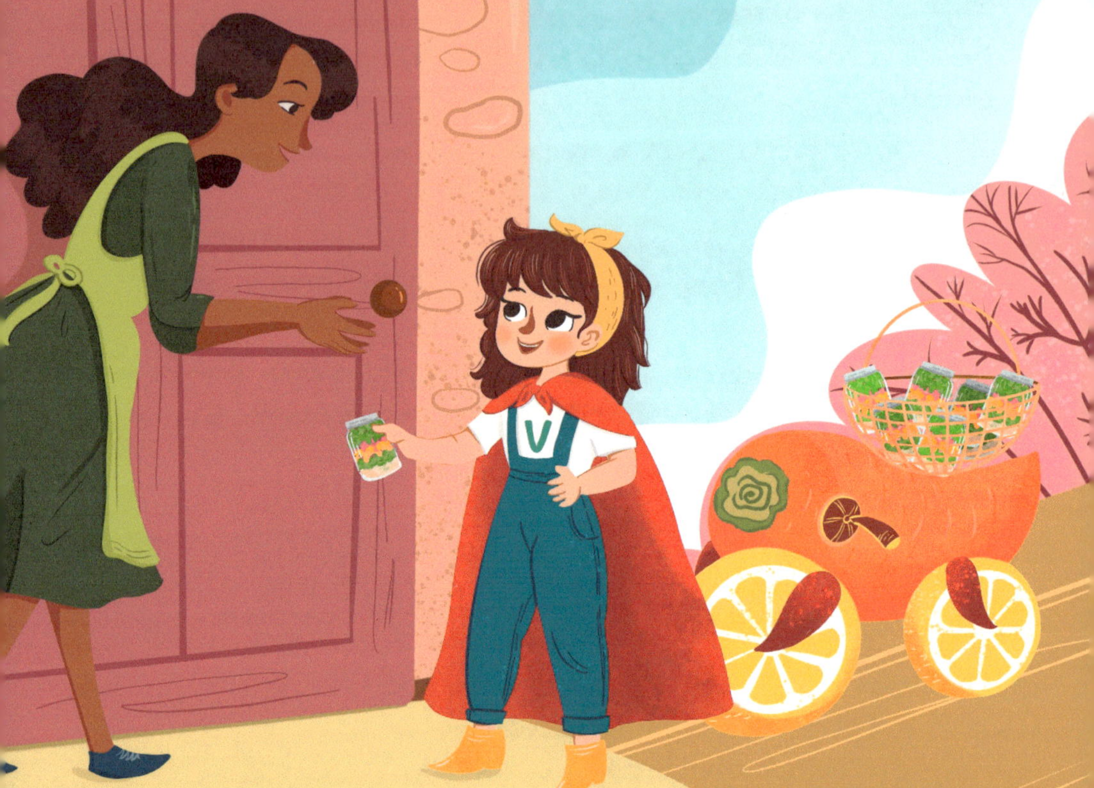

Quantities for this recipe are all based on your preference!

Ingredients:

- 1 mason jar with lid
- raw broccoli
- red grapes
- garbanzo beans (rinsed)
- sunflower seeds
- dried cranberries (or raisins)
- shredded carrots
- Dressing of choice

(dressing idea: 2 tbsp balsamic vinigrette, 3 tbsp tahini, 1 tbsp water)

*Salad jars are all about layering your ingredients! Follow my guide, or layer in any order you prefer!

Steps:

1. Chop your broccoli into little bite-sized florets and drop a handful into the jar.
2. Cut your grapes in half and place a handful into the jar.
3. Add in some cooked garbanzo beans.
4. Add shredded carrots to the jar.
5. Add sunflower seeds and dried cranberries. (Substitute cranberries with raisins, if necessary!)
6. Add dressing of your choice to the top.
7. Seal the lid of your jar and SHAKE it up really well! Taste-test it.. add a bit of salt, if desired. Shake some more! Open & Enjoy.

Note:
Salad in a jar can be made with any salad ingredients! Just layer the chopped ingredients, add your dressing and shake, shake shake!

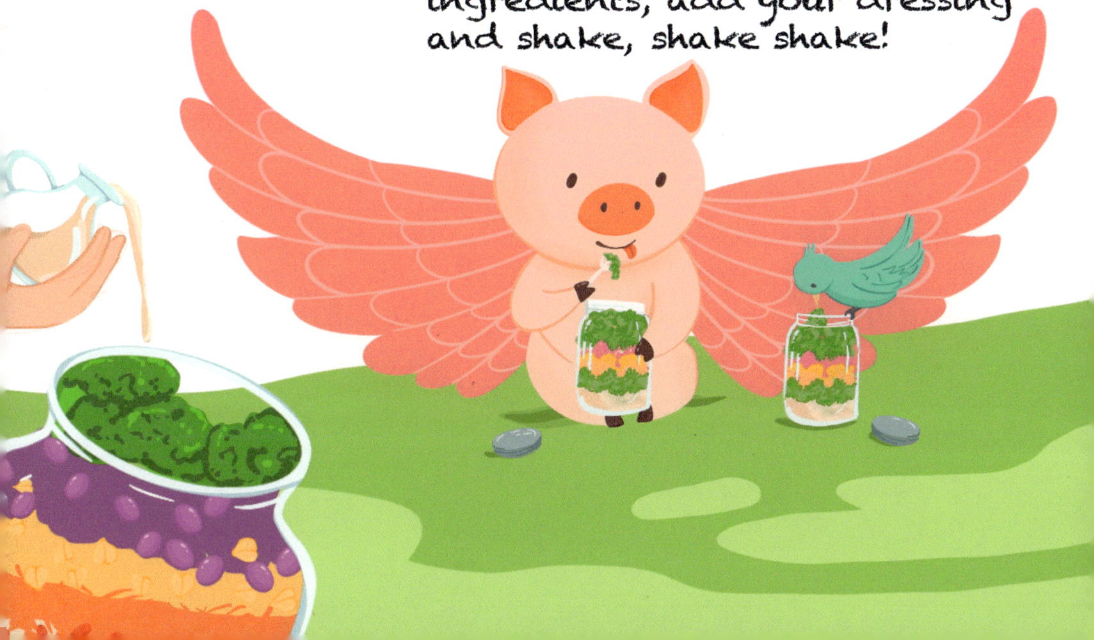

Stuffed Bell Peppers

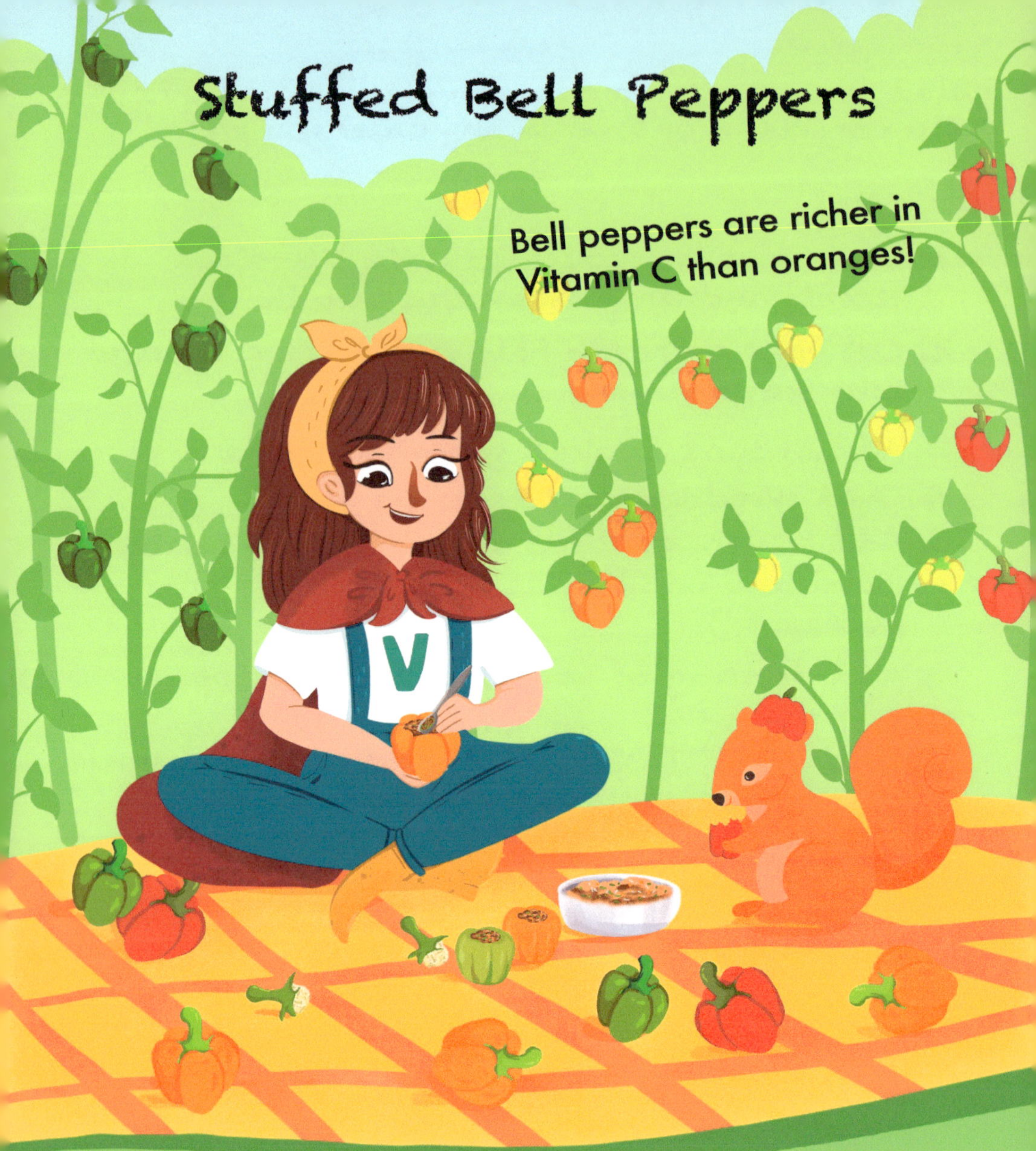

Ingredients:

- Bell Peppers (mini or full sized)
- 1/2 cup of Brown Rice (or quinoa) cooked
- 1/4 cup of Black Beans (cooked/rinsed)
- 1/4 cup of Sweet Corn
- 1 heaping tbsp of Hummus
- 1/2 tablespoon of Lime Juice
- 1 Green Onion
- Salt & Pepper to taste

Steps:

1. In a mixing bowl, add your quinoa or rice, beans and corn.

2. Chop your green onion into little bits and add it to the mixing bowl along with your hummus and lime juice.

3. Mix it all up! It should be a thick and creamy mixture. Taste-test it before adding salt.. It may not need salt at all, depending on the hummus used.

4. Slice the top off your bell pepper(s). Gently hollow out the inside of the pepper, if needed.

5. Using a spoon, stuff the bell pepper with the mixture. Enjoy this raw, or bake for 10-12 minutes at 350 degrees.

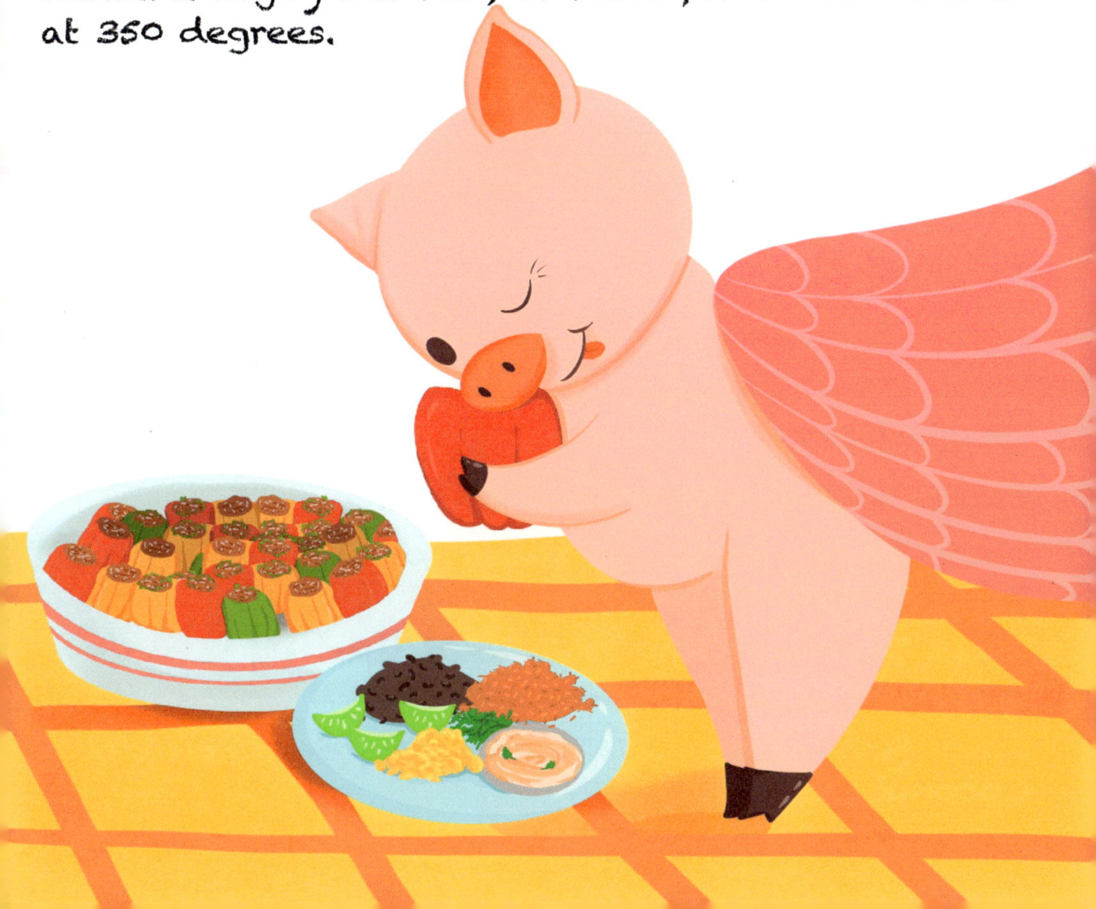

Fruit Pizza

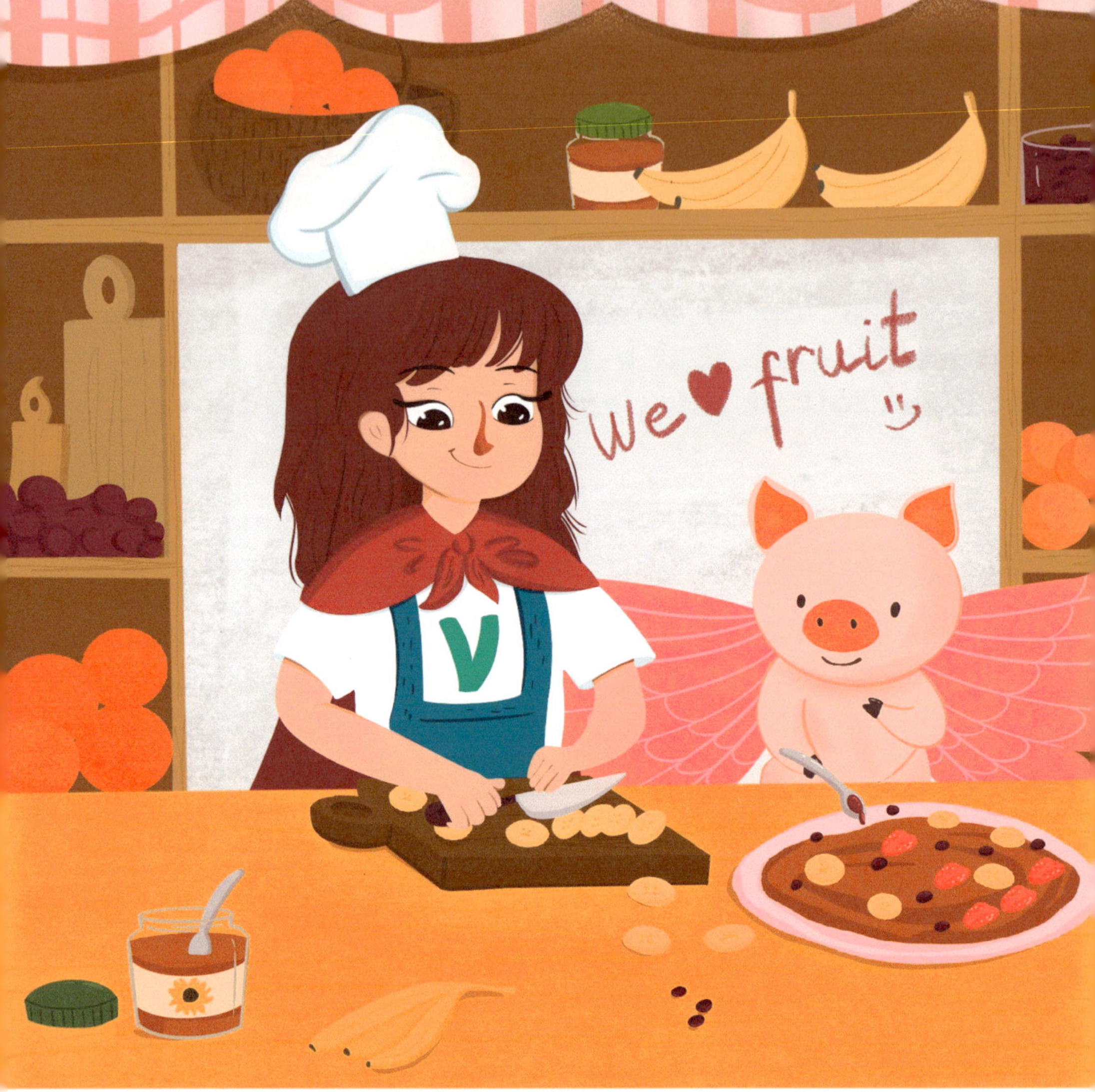

Ingredients:

Pizza Base- Dry Rice Cake or Waffle

Pizza Sauce- Sunflower butter (or any seed or nut butter of your choice!)

Pizza Toppings- Any fruit you'd like! My favorite is banana, strawberry and kiwi slices.

Pizza Seasonings- Chia Seeds, Hemp Seeds and/or Coconut Flakes

Steps:

1. Spread a layer of sunflower butter (or nut butter) all over the base of your pizza.
2. Chop your toppings and add them to the pizza!
3. Sprinkle on your seasonings. Enjoy!

** Bonus Fruit Recipe! **

Chia Seed Pudding Parfait:

1. Add 4 tablespoons of chia seeds into 1 cup of plant-based milk.
2. Add 1/2 a tablespoon of maple syrup. Sprinkle in some cinnamon (optional). Stir it well and allow it to set for 2 hours or overnight. The chia seeds will expand, taking on a thick pudding-like texture. If it seems too liquidy after a few hours, add more chia!
3. Once the consistency is right, add your chopped fruit toppings plus granola, if desired. Healthy and delicious!

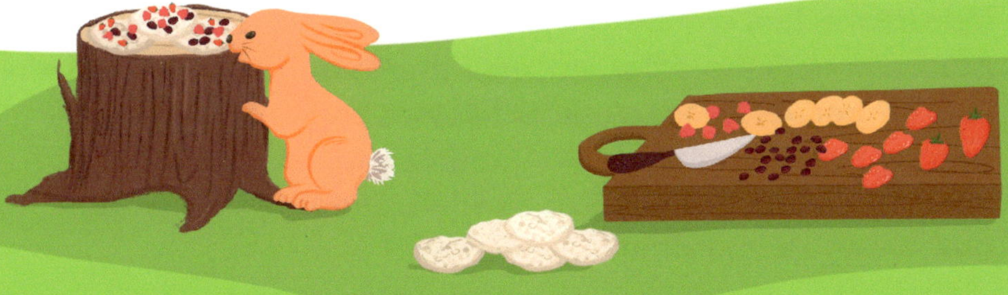

A few more of Veggie Vero's favorites:

Heart of Palm Ceviche

Ingredients- Hearts of palm (rinsed), lime juice, coconut milk (canned full fat), tomato, cucumber (remove skin), cilantro, red onion, sea kelp flakes (for ocean taste), salt and pepper.

Instructions- Chop it all up, mix together in a bowl and serve with your favorite tortilla chips! Sea kelp is optional, but highly recommended for taste and nutrition. You can substitute with Nori sheets, if needed, by chopping them up into small bits. Start with a small amount of coconut milk & lime juice, then adjust to taste.

Pumpkin Squash & Chickpea Soup

Ingredients- Organic pumpkin puree, vegetable stock, coconut milk (canned, full fat), butternut squash and/or acorn squash, garbanzo beans, carrots, onion, salt, pepper, garlic chives, pumpkin seeds.

Instructions- Slice open your squash, drizzle with olive oil, and place in the oven to bake until tender. Combine all liquid ingredients in a pot to simmer along with the chickpeas, onion, and garlic chives. Once the squash is tender, remove any skin, chop it up and toss in the pot with liquids. Stir and taste-test. Add salt and pepper as needed. In the last 3 minutes of cooking, you can add a handful of spinach or your favorite greens into the pot. (This is optional. Personally, I love wilted greens inside of soup!) After serving in a bowl, top it off with pumpkin seeds!

Flavorful Cranberry Sauce

Ingredients- Fresh cranberries, oranges (or pure orange juice), dates, maple syrup, coconut shreds

Instructions- Boil cranberries until soft. Place in a blender or food processor with the dates, coconut shreds and orange juice. Pulse until desired texture is achieved. If you prefer a lumpy texture, add some un-blended (boiled) cranberries to your mixture. Taste-test and add maple syrup as needed. Dates are a natural sweetener, so you shouldn't need a lot of maple.

Spring Rolls (or Autumn Rolls!)

Ingredients- Rice paper wraps, water, veggies of your choice! For Spring rolls, I recommend carrots, cucumber, bell pepper, purple cabbage and *special sauce.
For Autumn rolls, I recommend cooked sweet potato, apple slices, cooked beets, and some butter lettuce, topped with special sauce and sprinkled with cinnamon.
***Ingredients for sauce** (This is a go-to sauce for many recipes) tahini, maple syrup, coconut aminos, & toasted sesame oil.

Instructions- Chop veggies into long vertical strips. Line them up onto the dry rice paper wrap, being careful not to crack the wrap. Drizzle your sauce on top. Now it's time to wet the rice paper, which will soften it and allow it to roll. To wet the wrap, you can use fresh water in a spray bottle, you can brush the water on with a baster brush, or use a wet napkin to gently rub the water on. My preferred method is the spray bottle! Give it about 90 seconds to really soften. If it's still not soft enough, add more water. Roll it up and enjoy!

Buddha Bowl

Ingredients- Quinoa (and/or brown rice), garbanzo beans, broccoli, sweet potato, purple carrots, sunflower seeds (or any seeds of your choice), dressing of your choice!

Instructions- Scoop your cooked grains into a serving bowl. Add a few spoonfuls of cooked garbanzo beans directly on top of the grains. If you'd like to create "rows" of toppings, add the garbanzo beans in a row, leaving space for the next ingredients. Chop your cooked sweet potato and add it to the bowl. Chop up your broccoli florets and add to the bowl. These can be cooked or raw. Chop and add the purple carrot (or any color, I just love the look of purple!) Sprinkle some sunflower seeds over top. Drizzle with your favorite dressing and enjoy!

Create Your Own Recipe!

Title: ______________________________

Ingredients: ______________________________

____

____

____

____

Instructions: ______________________________

____

____

____

____

____

____

____

____

Create Your Own Recipe!

Title: ______________________________________

Ingredients: ________________________________

____

____

____

____

Instructions: _______________________________

____

____

____

____

____

____

____

Made in the USA
Monee, IL
05 November 2026

67378939R00019